101 Tips Media and Marketing for Salon Owners Stylists and Managers

Nanette Miner
with Gino Moncada

BVC Publishing
Bristol, CT USA

101 Media and Marketing Tips for Salon Owners, Stylists and Managers

By Nanette Miner
with Gino Moncada

Published by:
BVC Publishing
P O Box 1819
Bristol, CT 06011
USA

Copyright © 2001 by BVC Publishing
ISBN 0-9650666-4-9
$9.95

Attention Professional Organizations and Trade Associations: Quantity discounts are available on bulk purchases (10 or more) of this book for educational purposes, fund raising, or gift giving. For more information please contact:
BVC Publishing at 1-888-282-4165

Table of Contents

⊰ Preface ⊱

Why a book on marketing for salon owner, stylists, and managers?
Because of the reality of every stylist – you <u>are</u> your business. And
you're on a limited budget. Every tip provided in this book keeps
those two realities in mind. When choosing which tips to include
and which to leave out, the included tips had to meet four criteria:

1. They cannot take forever to accomplish. Usually idea to
    fruition can be accomplished within a week - many times
    within a day; some take less than an hour.

2. They cannot cost more than $500 to implement - most cost
    under $100.

3. They must be relationship oriented so that once you attract
    a new customer you keep him.

4. They must be professional in appearance and execution.

This book is intended to help all stylists and salon
owners/managers to establish visibility and credibility, and to
enhance marketability. As a bonus, increased sales will come.

◄ NETWORKING ►

Tip #1   How to Network

Networking is unequivocally the most valuable business tool you can possess. Networking allows you to make potential business connections in a non-sales way.

Three keys to becoming a successful networker, are:

1. Join associations (professional, community) and become active. Volunteer. Don't wait for "them" to come to you. Walk right up to the president or the chair of a committee and ask, "How can I help?"

2. When faced with a room full of strangers, act is if you are the host/hostess. Introduce yourself to others; introduce your new acquaintance to others. This becomes much easier when you've taken step one; now you can approach people and say, "Hi, I'm Chris. I'm on the membership committee…"

3. Encourage others to speak about themselves. Express an active interest in others. Don't dominate the conversation with what you do – it can come across as a sales pitch.

Tip #2   Chambers of Commerce

Chambers of Commerce are one of the best ways to meet the "movers and shakers" in your community. Network with other managers, salons, and CEO's from the businesses in your area. If you live in an area that doesn't have a large enough business community to support a chamber, join the chamber of commerce from a neighboring community. Many people mistakenly believe that if the work in X-town they can only join the X-town chamber. Not true! Pick that association that's going to do the most for you.

Tip #3   Professional Associations

There are thousands of professional associations out there, from retailers to advertising agents, to salespeople and manufacturers … the list goes on and on. It's easy to waste money by joining too many associations or the wrong ones. Be sure you thoroughly understand the association's purpose and the benefits of joining. Be selective, start with two or three associations and visit a few times as a guest. Get a feel for the members, the types of programs, and the benefits your membership would give you. You will learn much about running and marketing your business from your professional associations such at The Salon Associations (TSA) and The National Cosmetology Associations (NCA) as well as local professional associations such as the Exchange Club.

Tip #4   Professional Associations, cont.

Belonging to a professional association doesn't magically bring you business. Being able to state, "Member of _____" rarely causes the new customer to say, "That's why I chose you as my salon." Belonging to your professional association – and being active as a volunteer – does assist you in becoming well known in your business community. You will find that your business colleagues will refer business to you when it is something they cannot provide themselves (such as coloring specialists or spa services).

Tip #5   Non-Professional Associations

There are just as many non-professional associations as there are professional associations. Individuals and business people from all walks of life join for the networking opportunities. Associations for the self-employed abound. Check your local newspaper for notices of meetings of the Exchange Club, Lions Club, Rotary Club or small-business organizations. The more people who know you and know what you do – the more opportunity there is for business to be referred to you.

Tip #6   Bridal Fairs

Bridal fairs are a great place to promote your business. Typically the fair organizers will only allow a limited number of competing businesses to display their wares (you may find you are the only salon at the fair). Be sure to have lots of freebies and perhaps a drawing for services to attract attendees to your booth (you could have a drawing for an item, but the idea is to get people into your salon, later). Don't just concentrate on attracting people to your booth; during slow periods, walk the floor and visit the other booths, introduce yourself and leave behind some freebies. <u>Everyone</u> needs your services.

Tip #7 Fairs and Expos

If you find the cost of taking your own booth at a bridal expo or fair to be too high, buddy-up with a complimentary merchant and share the booth space. For instance, you do hair and your buddy does accessories. You have now doubled your ability to attract people to your booth while cutting your costs in half.

Tip # 8 Presentations to Civic Clubs

Civic clubs, such as the Women's Club or Newcomer's Club are always looking for speakers for their weekly or monthly meetings. You might even host the monthly meeting at your salon. Talk about and demonstrate things that the attendees could do at home to make themselves look and feel better. Notice the meeting announcements in the newspaper and contact the person who is given as the club-contact. You'll find they rarely turn down an offer of a speaker. This format allows you to contact and impress 15 or more people at a time.

Tip #9   Fundraisers

Cut-a-thons or similar events are not only fun, they also raise money for a good cause and they get your name in the limelight in association with a worthy cause. You can't buy advertising that gets you better exposure than the exposure you will receive from having people flock to your salon for services in association with a charitable cause.

Tip #10   Charitable Donations

Always offer to do the hair and makeup for local non-profit or charitable organizations that have the need. For instance, the "Miss Fall Festival" pageant might be held in your town or a nearby town, or the senior high might be holding a spring fashion show. Of course, be sure that your name and location are displayed on a banner or in printed material if there are programs. Associations who are receiving free services will rarely begrudge you a free promotional message.

Tip # 11   Referral Cards

Word of mouth advertising is the best advertising you can receive. You have a large sales force in the customers that already come to your salon. Print up a supply of referral cards and give them to your present customers. Ask them to refer their friends, family, and business associates by writing their name on the card and giving it to the referral. For every five cards that come into the salon from the same individual, offer them 10% off a service of their choice, or a free product, or perhaps a free service (they have brought in a couple of hundred dollars worth of business, after all).

Tip #12   Friends and Family Discount

You may find the "friends and family discount" to be the only promotion you need! Give your friends and family members (and *their* friends and family members) a price-cut on services if they come during your typically slow periods. Offering 10% off or $10 off your services is enough incentive for many, many individuals to bring their business to you.

Tip #13   Samples

If you receive free samples from your vendors, be sure to staple your business card to them before you distribute them. Think of unusual ways to distribute them. A basket on the counter of a neighboring business? At PTA meetings?

Tip #14   Competition? What Competition?

Don't see your competitors as competitors – view them as collaborators. What do you provide that they don't, and vice versa? How can you help your customers by introducing them to your competitor and how can s/he do the same? Some ideas for collaborators are: massage services, nails, skin care, plastic surgeons, health clubs. Work out a mutually beneficial agreement to provide those products or services that your competitors cannot, and vice versa.

Tip #15   Ask What You Can Do

There is a lot of truth in the saying, "It is better to give than to receive." When entering into any networking opportunity: professional association, chamber of commerce, spouse's company picnic – do not think of yourself and what you can get through our interaction with others, but, rather, think of what you can give to others. You'll find that what you give frequently comes back to you exponentially.

◄ GIFTS, GIMMICKS & GIVEAWAYS ►

Tip #16　　You're a Lifesaver!

When someone does something you are thankful for or has gone above the call of duty, send them a small, padded envelope with a roll of Lifesavers and a note that says:

"Thanks! You're a lifesaver!"

Tip #17　　Audio Tapes

Every person spends too much time in their car. Audio tapes are a great way to have a captive audience and promote your business as well. You can give your customers generic audio tapes such as nature sounds or comedy albums, or you may tape your own 20 minute "beauty update" every month or every quarter. Generic tapes can be purchased at bookstores or through audio book clubs. Give them to new clients as a thank you, "old" clients as a way to keep in touch, or give one to each of your clients at holiday time. Be sure one side of the tape has an audio label with your salon information!

Tip #18　　Video Tapes

Many people are unable to achieve the same look when doing their own hair that you are able to do for them in the salon. You might video tape yourself drying and styling their hair so that they can do it themselves at home. Charge a small fee ($5) or give the tape away. Be sure there is a label with your salon information!

Tip #19   And The Winner Is!

Hold a raffle. During the course of one-week give each customer ½ of a raffle ticket. Raffle tickets are inexpensive and can be purchased at any party supply store. At the end of the week choose a winner from the accumulated tickets. Be sure to have a big bowl and lots of eye-catching displays on the counter to collect the tickets. The prize doesn't have to be big – a mug, a product, or a free haircut. It makes your salon a fun place to visit and keeps customers coming back because they might win next time.

Tip #20   Compliments Of...

Put a flyer or specialty item (Post-It® note, pen) in the event bag of the school science fair, the local college's technology fair, or local business expo. It's cheaper than having your own booth, and you're assured that everyone who attends gets your marketing material.

Tip #21   Stick It!

Give away a funny or poignant Post-It® Note (something about a bad hair day, perhaps?). They can be purchased at all office supply stores, through catalogs, and through custom printers on the internet. When possible, have your notes custom printed with your salon name and contact information. Each time your customer uses the notes – she will think of you.

Tip #21   Giveaways

If you have a supply of product that isn't moving, package it with a more desirable item at half-price or as a giveaway. You may also special-purchase giveaway items such as combs, brushes, or nail files to give in combination with a product purchase from your salon. Customers always appreciate receiving something for free – no matter how small the item.

◄ DATABASES/MAILING LISTS ►

Tip #22　　Databases and Mailing Lists

Before you spend money purchasing a mailing list, investigate all of the free options that are available. For instance, the names and addressees of all homeowners in your town are public information and are available from the assessor's office.

Tip #23　　Target Your Mailings

If you choose to conduct mass mailings in your town or a surrounding area, be sure to target the mailing to people who can actually use and afford your services. Targeting will save you money by not sending promotions to individuals who would never respond. You may choose to target by neighborhood (the ones in your surrounding area) or income level (you know which areas in your town are pricier homes and which are not) or customer-type (families with children under the age of 12).

Tip # 24　　List Brokers

List brokers will help you to narrow down your choices regarding who you need to target, where they are likely to be found, and what they are likely to be interested in. The broker makes a commission by selling the list to you. It behooves the broker to sell you the list again, or to purchase a different list, so s/he will work hard for you. Think of the list broker as a consultant and use all of the services that s/he can give you.

Tip #25   One Time Use

You may not purchase a mailing list, you may only rent them. The list perpetually belongs to the list owner. Mailing list rentals run between 4 cents and 25 cents per name and allow you one time use. The list owner will "salt" the list with names that will return to him. In this way the list owner can be sure of your honesty in using the list only once. If they receive a second mailing from you – expect to be billed again.

Tip #26   Create Your Own List

The longer you are in business, the more contacts and customers you will collect. Before you rent somebody else's list, be sure to maximize the use of your own list. Have all new customers fill out an information form that includes their name, address, birth date (month/day; not year!), and e-mail address.

Tip #27   Birthday or Anniversary Mailings

Thank your customers for their business at least once yearly. Too many businesses send holiday cards - so it's easy to get lost in the volume. Consider, instead, sending a birthday card with an exclusive offer. Even more unique is an anniversary card on the date that the customer started frequenting your salon. When you have the new customer fill out an information sheet, be sure to have an area where they can mark "today's date."

Tip #28   E-mail Lists

Virtually everyone has e-mail access. E-mail newsletters or promotions are the most cost effective method of reaching your customers. It costs you nothing and allows you to be more consistent in your "mailings". Find an internet list management service so that administration of your growing e-mail list is as pain free for you as possible.

Tip #29   Exchange (or sell) Your List

You need to have a rather extensive personal list (5000+ names) before a list broker will represent you. But there are ways to use your list in your own community. If you refer your customers to non-competing, but complimentary businesses, why not use the lists those businesses have compiled in exchange for your list? Would the owner of the other business be willing to write a short letter of introduction so that your mailing is well received? If you sell your list, charge at least 25 cents per name – remember, this is a small and highly targeted list, and you are endorsing the person who is using it. It is worth the higher per-name price.

◄ INTERNET ►

Tip #30   Web Page Design

Consider this: do you have the time and the talent to design a web page yourself? If not, you'll need to hire someone to do it. Lots of people will <u>tell</u> you that they can design your web page. Make sure to see plenty of sample pages the designer has created for other businesses. Create as much of the content as you can. Remember, you're the expert in your business, the person you hire is expert in web design.

Tip #31   Web Page Hosting

In addition to having a web page designed, it must be hosted, or stored, on an internet server. Hosting services can range from $29 per month to over $100 per month depending on how much space you need, among other things. Consider whether or not you want to sell product or gift certificates via your web site; if so, you'll need a secure site, which will add to your monthly hosting expenses.

Many on-line services offer free space for web pages but may not be able to assist you when things go wrong, like a dedicated web hosting service will.

Tip #32   Market Your Services via Other Web Pages

Consider marketing your business via web pages other than your own. Your chamber of commerce may have a site or a "hometown news" site might exist for your town. Consider sponsoring the local senior center's web page or the pre-school's web page. Sponsorship or advertising on these pages will cost you from $25 to $100 per year and will be much less labor intensive than maintaining your own site. The added benefit is that these other sites will attract people who may never have found your business on their own because they weren't looking for a new salon.

Tip #33   Put Links to Other Sites on Yours

Most people are looking for information on the web. The more information you can provide the more your site is likely to be considered to be a destination spot for your customers and prospective customers. Link to product manufacturers so that customers can go direct to the manufacturer from your site, should they choose to do so. Be sure to include the product logo to reinforce the idea that customers can buy these products from you.

Tip #34   Gaining Web Site Exposure

The World Wide Web is destined to be as popular as television, and far more useful. Your web site will need to come to the top of the pile to be successful. You can achieve this through the use of key words that will attract customers. Your web designer should be able to submit your site to the search engines, as well as designing it for you. Be sure that you choose the key words since you best understand your business.

Tip #35   Domain Name

Your address on the web is as important as your business name, which you took considerable care in choosing. Having your own domain name makes it easy for customers to find your site and remember your web address.

It's getting more and more difficult to get a desirable domain name. Don't be surprised if your name is already in use by a salon miles and miles away. The situation will only worsen as time goes on. Even if you don't plan to start a web site for awhile, it's a good idea to register your domain name now so you don't "lose" it to someone else.

Tip #36   Promote Your Web Site Everyday

Be sure your web address is printed on your business cards, storefront window, smocks and products (for starters). The more customers can easily find your web address the more likely they are to visit your site.

◄ NEWSLETTERS ►

Tip #37   Make It Eye-Catching

You want your newsletter to be eye-catching. Unique design, sharp graphics, photos or cartoons, snappy name or title. Many software programs will allow you to make your newsletter yourself with a minimal amount of work.

Tip #38   Make It Eye-Catching, cont.

Hire a graphic artist to design a unique and colorful heading (the upper 1 to 2 inches of the page) and format for your newsletter. Use this design as a
master – take it to a print shop and have hundreds or thousands of the master made up. Each month (or quarter), format the newsletter on your computer, then run a stack of the header-paper through your laser printer. The newsletter will look as though it is custom printed each month and you save a lot of money by having the master duplicated en-mass.

Tip #39   Who to Mail To

Your newsletter will be best received by your current customers. They will be more likely to recognize your salon name and continue to read the contents of the newsletter. A newsletter sent to non-customers will most likely be perceived as junk mail.

Tip #40   Be Consistent

Determine how frequently you will mail your newsletter based on how consistent you can afford to be. A monthly mailing can be quite expensive. A quarterly newsletter might be more manageable. Another consideration is how much time you will have to devote to writing the newsletter. Monthly deadlines will creep up much faster than quarterly ones. If you start to send your newsletter monthly and then switch to a more infrequent pattern, you risk disappointing your customers. Better to figure out in advance, what type of schedule will allow you to be most consistent.

Tip #41   When to Mail

A quarterly newsletter will allow you to talk about "trends this season" in each issue and feature different products that are appropriate for the different seasons. At a minimum, send your newsletter twice per year.

Tip #42   Write When The Mood Strikes You

Too often you will have a good idea for inclusion in your next newsletter but when the time comes, you'll have forgotten what it was. Sit down and write out the <u>complete</u> text whenever you have a moment of inspiration. An alternative is to carry a small tape recorder with you to record your ideas when they hit. If you're able, write your newsletters three or six months in advance. This will allow you to carry through a theme from one newsletter to the next. Also, when the printing/mailing deadline approaches you won't feel as pressured.

Tip #43   Mailing Your Newsletter

Remember that database of businesses, customers, friends, and family you created? Start by mailing your newsletter to them. Ask for a referral in each newsletter – include an area that asks: "Do you know someone who would benefit from this newsletter? If so, please let us know who they are!" and include a space for them to fill out the contact's information. Set this area off with a border or some other eye-catching design.

Tip #44   Grab Their Attention

David Letterman made Top 10 Lists popular. Virtually everybody loves them.
We also love:

> The 5 Reasons Why…
>
> Seven Secrets Of…
>
> Three Things You MUST

The point is, numbered lists work. And they are easy to write. Questions also work well. Start your articles with compelling statements or questions such as:

> Do You Know Why Nearly Half of Our Customers…
>
> Recent Studies Reveal…

Tip #45   What To Include In The Newsletter

Use the newsletter to promote the business. Talk about all of the services that are offered, the importance of scheduling appointments (and canceling in a timely manner), and the convenience of your hours or location. Each newsletter might feature a different service provider and a short biography of that person. Great relationships are born, and continue, when the customers begin to think of their service providers as friends and family.

Tip #46   Create a Series or Theme

If you have a lot of information on a topic, create a series out of it. Reading a series is akin to reading a book – you can't wait to get to the next chapter to see what happens. Herald the next chapter by "teasing" your audience, "Next month we'll discuss..." Each month your newsletter could contain a column on hair, a column on nails, and a column on other services. To be more than "just a salon" to your customers, you might consider a column on health and nutrition news as well.

Tip #47   Postcard Newsletters

Postcards are so useful and versatile that the entire next chapter has been devoted to them. A postcard newsletter is sure to be read because it is short. It's also easy to write because...it is short. You must limit yourself to one or two major ideas because that is all that will fit. The recipient reads it before she even realizes it because it is easy to glance at a 3x5 card and absorb the information.

Tip #48   Email Newsletters

Email newsletters have advantages and disadvantages. One advantage is that it allows you to announce information to your customers on short notice and with little preparation. A disadvantage is that your customers may see it as another piece of junk cluttering their inbox. Do not distribute your email newsletter to anyone who did not sign up for it specifically (remember to ask for this information on your new customer information sheet). Keep your newsletter list on your work computer. If you keep it at home, then only <u>you</u> will be able to work on it, and you may come to resent it restricting your free time. If the newsletter is produced and distributed via the salon computer, you can sit down when an appointment is unexpectedly cancelled, or you can direct one of your employees to work on it under your supervision.

⊰ POSTCARDS ⊱

Tip #49   Postcards

A postcard has an immediate impact on the reader. You don't have to depend on the reader to open the envelope and discover what's inside.

Tip #50   Pre-formatted Postcards

Many office supply stores and stationary catalogs have pre-formatted postcard designs. They range from colored paper with borders, to photos of the world, money, or a handshake. They come in sheets of four and are easily fed through your laser printer. Cost is minimal: $7.00 - $10.00 per hundred depending on the design and the supplier. If you have a lot to say, purchase the "jumbo" 4x6 size which come two to a sheet.

Tip #51   Announcements

Postcards are a fast, easy, economical way to make announcements to your customer base:

Nancy Smith has joined our staff...

We have moved...

Now! Open until 7:00 on Thursday AND Friday!

We will be conducting a cut-a-thon at...

Announcing Product Clearance Specials!

Tip #52   Surveys

Thinking about changing your business in some way and wondering what your customer's will think of the change? Postcard surveys are easy to complete and take virtually no time at all. Keep the questions and answers simple: yes/no, rank 1-5; put an "x" next to the top three...

Mail to your customer base, or hand to customers when you see them and ask them to mail or fax them back.

Tip #53   Create Events

Use postcards to celebrate the number of years you've been in business.

> *Our 1st Anniversary Celebration!*
>
> *Happy Birthday ... to us!*
>
> *We're proud to have served the community for nine years.*

It's important to stay in touch with your customers as much as possible. Celebrating your yearly anniversary is a great reason to make contact.

Tip #54   Custom Postcards

You can create a customized, full color, postcard just for your business. Include your logo, your staff's picture, your storefront, your company colors – all the things that make your salon unique and recognizable. Use the custom postcards as you would the custom-designed newsletter.

Tip #55   "We've Missed You"

Send a postcard to those customers who haven't made an appointment in 60 or 90 days, telling them they've been missed and you'd like to see them at your salon again. Offer a "Welcome Back" discount.

A neat variation on this idea is the well-known, pink, "While You Were Out" memo. Personalize it to the recipient's attention. Include the stylist's name, salon name, and phone number. Add a brief message about something they've missed by not visiting recently, such as a product sale or new services that have been added. Be sure to check off the "Please Call" or "Wants To See You" box.

◄ IN PRINT ►

Tip #56   Leverage Your Expertise

Don't doubt your level of expertise by thinking, "Oh, everybody knows that." Everybody does not know what you know, and you'd be wise to leverage your expertise into profitable PR. Write a Top 10 List for your profession (example: 10 Ways to Keep Your Hair Healthy During Summer). Create an exciting article title, "Why _____ Never Works" (example: Why Do-It-Yourself Hot Oil Treatments Don't Work). You've spent years amassing your knowledge – use it to your benefit in newspaper articles and/or advertisements.

Tip #57   Create Ads That Look Like Articles

Most people are inclined to believe an article in a newspaper before an advertisement. The philosophy is that an article is 'newsworthy' and factual. You can create your ad to look and read just like a news article – quote 'expert sources' and include a picture. Be sure to write ADVERTISEMENT across the top in bold print. You can put the word ADVERTISEMENT in the upper right or left corner and make it slightly smaller than the type you are using for your article/ad.

Tip #58   Regular Monthly Columns

Virtually every professional association has a monthly or bi-monthly newsletter. And since most of these organizations are strictly staffed by volunteers – they are desperate for any help they can get! Write an article or a series of articles as a service to the organization. Of course, be sure your name and salon name and contact information are included in each article. Target female-oriented associations such as Women In Transportation or the National Association of Executive Assistants. Or, if you're particularly daring, target men's organizations and stress how men-friendly your salon is.

Tip #59   Leverage the Coverage You've Already Attained

Once you've been published in 3-4 newsletters or journals, make sure your by-line reads, "Pam Smith owns *A New You Salon* and writes frequently for xxx, xxx, and xxx." Now you're beginning to look like an industry expert!

Tip #60   Submit "Happenings" to Trade Magazines and Local Newspapers

Once you've conducted or participated in a charitable event, make a short press release to be distributed to your trade magazines and local newspapers (don't forget the small, once-a-week newspapers as well). Briefly state who benefited and how the salon participated (gave money, provided services, sponsored someone).

Publishing these notices in your trade magazines makes your salon attractive to future and potential stylists. The newspapers may publish your item to help fill space and participating in a charitable event can only reflect well on your salon. Each audience will think, "This salon believe in helping people."

Tip #61   Booklets

A booklet is an excellent marketing tool. Books give you credibility as well as a side-line income to your regular business. Offer booklets for sale at the counter or at special events where the salon is appearing. Two to three dollars is sufficient to entice people to brush up on techniques or learn new ones (example: Three New Up-Do's For Prom and Wedding Season). There are fairly cheap computer programs that allow you to first create the booklet in your own word processing package, then transform it into a side-by-side booklet, a three-fold brochure/booklet, or all sorts of other configurations.

Tip #62   Internet Sites

You can entice people to visit your salon by writing compelling and useful articles or columns that are published on other people's web sites. For example, a closet organizer could use an article titled: "Now That You've Made Over Your Closet, What About You?" A home re-modeler could use the same type of article. An herbal supplements vendor could use an article titled: "Taking Care of the Inside _and_ the Outside."

Try not to sell them but rather give good, useful information. The fact that you are so generous with your knowledge will "sell" them just the same.

◄ RADIO AND TV ►

Tip #63   Talk About What You Know

There are more than 1,000 daily talk shows in the US. In addition, every local morning show uses guests in one way or another. With the addition of morning and drive time radio shows, there is potential for 6,000 FREE media appearances each day. Surely you have something worthwhile to say about your profession that can fill 6-10 minutes.

Tip #64   Capitalize on Events or Seasons

You may find your marketability for radio appearances is limited to certain events or seasons, such as "wedding season," New Year's Eve or Holiday looks, or "Getting Ready for Summer." That's OK. Just don't lose the opportunity to capitalize on when the stations can use you. Give yourself enough planning time to execute your promotion during your busy seasons – the promotions can help carry you through the slumps that follow.

Tip #65   How to Find Radio Shows

You can search for radio stations in your area via the internet. Your topic is one that everyone is interested in and can use, so you won't be limited by the station's format. Approach the producer of each show (call first to find out that person's name). Be sure to contact the station a week to 10 days in advance so they can plan for your appearance. Any sooner and your pitch will be put in a pile somewhere and forgotten. If they ask for an interview – say yes! They will rarely try you again if you turn them down once. Accept any time and any location to participate in an interview – you can't afford to waste free advertising. Figure every minute you are on the air has saved you about $100 in advertising costs.

Tip #66   Radio Contacts in Your Area

Many radio hosts will have you on as a guest simply because you are a local "celebrity." To find out who to contact in your state, consult the Gale Directory of Publishing and Broadcast Media available at your local library; or use an internet search engine and type in "radio stations in (your state)."

Tip #67   What To Say When You Get There

One way to quickly stop being a radio or television guest is to flop. The hosts are looking for someone who is articulate and energetic. Three tips to being a better guest:

1.   Speak slowly and articulately. Speak in a relaxed manner, but not so relaxed that you are dropping the endings of words. Be aware of any verbal crutches you use such as "um," "well," or "you know."
2.   Prepare a list of question for the interviewer – nobody knows your business as well as you. Radio show hosts, especially, are doing twenty things at once. They greatly appreciate a list of questions that they can read that will make them sound as though they are quite familiar with you and your topic. An added benefit for you is that you are completely able to adress the questions since you created them!
3.   Prepare a few amusing, interesting, or poignant stories, anecdotes, or quotes to illustrate your points. Although you may have a serious message to share, remember that the host's job is to entertain the audience and keep them tuned in.

Tip #68   Create a Media Event

Local television news stations are always looking for "filler" stories. Create a media event and invite the media. Make a donation of surplus products to a local homeless shelter. Sponsor a little league team or soap box derby competition. Host an ice cream social to kick off the junior high science fair. Think of an event that the local media is likely to be intrigued by and want to share with their viewers.

Tip #69　　　Be Ready, Willing, and Able

If you are a popular guest, you will frequently receive requests to appear at unusual hours – 6:00 am or 12 midnight. You'll also receive last minute requests when a scheduled guest cancels. Don't be finicky. Say yes. No PR is bad PR, as they say.

Tip #70　　　Local Cable Access

Local cable access stations are always looking for shows – especially ones that would interest a wide-variety of viewers. Host a makeover show on local cable-access – live in your salon! You might even create a weekly series of makeovers – men, women, new-moms, elderly...the possibilities are endless. If you start a weekly show you'll end up being producer, crew, and haircutter. Be sure you have enough friends who are willing to work as camera people or studio engineers. This might be a great opportunity to spotlight different stylists in your salon as well.

◄ OTHER GREAT IDEAS! ►

Tip #71   Gift Certificates

Give gift certificates to your customers as holiday gifts. Use them to lure customers away from your competitors. Distribute them as anniversary gifts in thanks for your customer's patronage over the last year. Gift certificates can be purchased, pre-formatted and blank, from all office supply stores and paper catalogs.

Tip #72   Motivational Words

When creating news releases or promotional items, there are a few words that generate immediate interest:
- ∇   Free
- ∇   New
- ∇   Win
- ∇   Easy
- ∇   Introducing
- ∇   Save
- ∇   Guaranteed

Tip #73   Letters of Introduction

You might as well be the first person to introduce yourself to newcomers in the area. While services like Welcome Wagon® and Welcome Neighbor® can do that for you, for a fee, you can do it just as easily yourself by following the real estate transactions that are published on a weekly basis in your local paper.

Tip #74   PS

Research has shown that when sending a direct mail letter, a PS at the bottom garners more attention than the entire body of the letter. If you are going to promote your business or services via letters of introduction to potential customers, make something up – anything – and include it in a PS. Example: PS: Tuesday is our slowest day – call now for an appointment!

Tip #75   Survey New Customers

Your follow-up contact with a new customer is just as important as your initial contact with that customer. Within 3-5 days of a new customer's visit, survey them about the services they received. Included a postage-paid reply card so that they feel free to respond anonymously and are honest with you about how you can improve or what you are doing well. You may include a discount coupon with the survey so that they feel slightly more obligated to complete and return it.

Tip #76   Multiple Offer/Direct Mail Packs

Every week you receive an envelope filled with coupons and offers from merchants in your area. This may be an economical way to advertise your business. The cost of postage is divided among all the merchants who are participating in the mailing. Be careful not to include a coupon in each mailing or you will soon discover that your customers wait for the coupon and don't come in otherwise.

Tip #77   Thank You Product

You probably receive many sample packets from your distributors. If you don't receive them for free, or you don't get enough free samples, purchase a few dozen and hand them out to each customer who visits in a particular week. This is a great way to introduce new products you are beginning to carry. Be sure that whomever is handing out the free samples (you or perhaps a receptionist) has a "sales pitch" to go along with the product. You may announce the free samples in a newsletter in advance of the promotion, so that customers purposely schedule their appointments during that week.

Tip #78   Internet Coupons

One of the keys to a good website is to have your customers return again and again. You might try offering a different coupon each month – for product that isn't selling well, or a service that you are just introducing (skin care, nail care). The coupons should only be available via your website – that way customers will be sure to visit each month to find out what the coupon is for, whether or not they take advantage of the coupon that month.

Tip #79   Sponsor Your Own Community Event

Are you an avid golfer or basketball player? Gather 20 of your friends together and create your own tournament. Collect entry fees and donate a portion to the local boys and girls club, battered women's shelter, or hospice. Be sure to get the local media to come and take pictures of you giving the check to the charity.

Tip #80   Collaborate

Don't view your competitors as competitors – view them as collaborators. What do you provide that they don't, and vice versa? How can you help your customers by introducing them to your competitor and how s/he do the same for you? Do you need a shorter lead time than your competitor? Can you provide smaller quantities or make house calls? Work out a mutually beneficial agreement to provide those products or services that you cannot provide, but your competitor can.

Tip #81   Create a Salon Services Club

People are compelled to continue to use your services or buy your products when they are working toward a reward at the end. You can easily create a card by buying business cards at the stationary store and printing them with "12th haircut free" or "FREE _____ with purchase of 10." Simply add numbers to the card and hole-punch a new number each time the customer makes a qualifying purchase. These cards can also be created by custom-printers for a relatively low fee. Having a printer create them for you will make them more long-lasting as well, because you can have the cards printed on coated or heavy-stock paper.

Tip #82   Flashback

During slow business periods, plan a "Flashback" event to attract business. Roll back your prices to the 50's, 60's or 70's. Make it a one-day or one-week event. For added fun, ask your staff to dress appropriately for the era. Make sure to announce your event to radio stations, TV stations, newspapers, and community events – and don't forget your storefront window!

Tip #83   Unusual Advertising

Don't forget unusual sources of advertising: church bulletins, senior citizen newsletters, your health club or alumni newsletter, programs for the high school concert or your niece's dance recital. Frequently you are able to place a monthly ad in these bulletins for less than $100 (sometimes that's the price for the whole year!). An added bonus is that your competition is rarely visible in these unusual venues.

Tip #84   New Client Phone Calls

In today's era of impersonal service, when most people just feel like a number, the time invested in calling new clients will make you stand out from the completion. Two or three days after their first appointment, call new customers to ask if they liked their service, if they are able to style their hair on their own, and if they would like to schedule their next appointment at your regularly suggested interval of 6/5/4 weeks. Be sure your call is more about service and satisfaction than sales – the sale will come if you put emphasis on the service.

Tip #85   Pro Bono Work

Pro bono work is particularly effective when starting a new business or when your business needs a burst of activity. Let all the charitable organizations in your area know that your salon is available for in-house or on-site pro bono work. Offer services to homeless shelters, welfare-to-work organizations, hospices, pageants, fashion shows and other community events. Eventually you may need a way to "qualify" requests because you will receive so many! Charitable work always reflects well on your business. Be sure to use PR with this technique.

Tip #86   Persistence

Persistence is key. The typical sales pitch is ignored or resisted six times before the prospective client is ready to purchase or use your services. Keep up your marketing efforts on a regular basis – dependent on your budget. Monthly? Bi-monthly? Quarterly? Whatever schedule you choose, be sure the customer can count on you during that period of time.

Tip #87   Accept Credit Cards

Credit cards can boost your sales by as much as 20%. The person that only has $50 in their pocket for a $45 haircut won't buy $20 worth of product if you don't accept credit cards. The fees charged by credit card companies are nominal compared with the increased sales you will be able to generate.

Tip #88   Print Advertising

If you place ads in newspapers, flyers, or magazines, be sure to vary the ad's content or angle frequently. A new ad will attract a different group of people each time it appears. Pictures are very attractive to readers. Try a picture of a style one month, your staff another, and a community event held at your salon the third month.

Tip #89   News Releases

Try not to let any significant event slip by without a press release announcing it to your local news sources. Not every one will be picked up, of course, but the more attempts you make, the more likely it is you will appear in print. News releases should be double spaced with two-inch margin at top and bottom and one-and-a-half inch margins on the left and right. The news release should answer the questions: who, what, where, when and why?

Tip #90   Joint Mailings

If you are planning on a direct-mail campaign to your customer base, search out a complimentary service to share the mailing with you. You can fit four single sheets of 8.5 x 11 paper in an envelope for the same first class postage stamp. You could combine services with a masseuse, chiropractor, health-food store or other service that makes people feel better about themselves.

Tip #91   Vendor Malls/Trade Shows

Many professional associations, chambers of commerce, and community groups hold yearly showcases for their member's products and services.   Because they are locally produced they are relatively inexpensive and allow you to make a person-to-person connection with your target market. Consider on-the-spot services you can offer such as bang trimming, nail buffing, or up-do's.

Tip #92   Headshots

Why use the headshot posters you get from manufacturers and vendors? Make your own! When a stylist (or client) is particularly pleased with the work done, take a few photos to showcase the work. You can spotlight a stylist of the month in a display case at the entrance to your salon, showing 3-5 different looks that stylist created. Of course, include a photo and bio of the stylist as well. When a bio includes personal information about the stylist, such as *"she lives in ourtown with her husband and four dogs,"* people feel a much more personal connection with that individual.

Tip #93   Multiple Phone Lines

Nothing is more annoying to the customer than to get a busy signal when they are trying to give you business. Be sure to have at least two and preferably three lines in your salon that roll from one to another (your local phone service can set up "busy rollover" for you). In addition to the receptionist, there should be a designated person to answer the second and third line in case the receptionist is tied up with a customer. The designated person need do nothing more than answer the phone and explain that the receptionist is assisting a customer at the moment and will be with them shortly.

Tip #94   Stickers and Stamps

It is expensive to print stationary, business cards and brochures. Whenever possible make these items as generic as possible and update them with stickers or custom-stamps you buy at the local office supply store. Custom stamps can be made for as little as $4.00 and as much as $25.00 –far cheaper than having your materials reprinted when you add a new stylist or service. Other ideas for stickers and stamps: anniversary, reminder, thank you.

Tip # 95   Video Tape

Make an "infomercial" about your salon with your own video camera. Feature services you provide, conduct interviews with stylists, and ask willing customers to provide testimonials. Make it fun and eye appealing. Run the video on a small TV/VCR combination in the waiting area of your salon.

Tip #96   Business Cards

Make sure each of your stylists has business cards and carries them with them at all times. When giving out business cards, give three, with the line:
> *One for you, one for a friend, and one for the fridge.*

Tip #97   Customer Feedback

You can spend a lot of money on advertising and marketing and not accomplish much in the end. Why? Because paid advertising is paid advertising and the customer knows that you're crowing about yourself. Ask your clients to provide feedback about the services they received at your salon (both the service they paid for and the people-side of the service). With your customer's permission, use these comments in advertising, postcards, and your salon newsletter.

Tip #98   Guarantee Your Work

An unconditional guarantee gives your customers confidence in both your work and your professionalism. You don't have to refund their money, but do guarantee the quality of your workmanship. If a customer is unhappy with the service they received, offer to do whatever it takes to fix it within 48 hours. This is another good reason to call your customers to ask if they are pleased with the services they received.

Tip #99   Hotel/Motel Directories

Hotels and motels usually have in-room directories of services that are in the area. Many times there is no charge to be listed in the directory because the hotel sees it as an added service they are providing to their guests. Especially target extended stay hotels and hotels that cater to wedding parties who might need their beauty needs attended to at the last minute. As an extra convenience, you may offer in-room service and/or evening appointments for these guests.

Tip #100   How Did You Hear of Us?

When you ask new customers to fill out an information sheet make sure you ask, *How did you hear of us*? This allows you to track how well your various promotional efforts are working, and keep up what works best.

Tip #101   Model Nights/Education Nights

Once a month offer Model Night or Education Night. Offer drastically reduced prices or even free services to customers who are willing to have a new technique practiced on them by one of your stylists. Be sure to take pictures during and after so that you can use them for promotional purposes both in the salon and in advertisements.

◄ RESOURCES ►

AUDIO CASSETTES

Amazon.com	www.amazon.com
Audio Books Direct	317-541-8920
Audio-Tech Business Books	800-776-1910

CREDIT CARD MERCHANTS

NOVUS	800-347-2000

DATABASES/ MAILING LISTS

ACT!	www.symantec.com
American List Council	800-403-1870 www.alclists.com
Avery Label Pro	800-252-8379 www.avery.com (free trial version)
Acxiom/Direct Media	www.acxiom.com
PCS Mailing Lists	800-532-5478
Dun & Bradstreet	www.dnb.com
Hugo Dunhill Mailing Lists	888-274-5734 www.hdml.com
InfoUSA/BusinessUSA	800-555-5335 www.SalesLeadsUSA.com www.infoUSA.com
Edith Roman	800-223-2194 www.edithroman.com

DIRECTORIES

National Trade and Professional Associations of the United States	Columbia Books Inc. 1212 New York Ave. NW Suite 300 Washington, DC 20005
Business Publications Rates and Data Directory	(check your local library)
Encyclopedia of Associations	Gale Research Co. Book Tower Detroit, MI 48277-0748

FOOD

A Southern Season	800-253-3663
Hershey's	800-544-1347
	www.hersheygifts.com
Wine Country Gift Baskets	800-394-0394
	www.giftprogram.com

GIFT CERTIFICATES

Paper Direct	800-272-7377
Viking Office Products	800-421-1222

GIFTS, GIMMICKS & GIVEAWAYS

Donut Boxes	800-851-1241
	www.donutbox.com
Successories	800-535-2773
Direct Promotions	800-444-7706
Viking Business Giveaways	800-421-1222
Oriental Trading	800-228-2269

INTERNET

Vision Technologies Inc.	Vti@vtinet.com
	www.vtinet.com
Zy Graphics	ww.zy.com
Download.com	www.download.com
The Free Site	www.thefreesite.com

NEWSLETTERS

Microsoft Publisher	www.microsoft.com/products/
PrintShop Publishing Suite	800-779-6000
	www.parsonstech.com
Newsletters and More	800-779-6000
	www.parsonstech.com

PHOTOS

Black and White Reproductions JEM Photo	412-621-0331 www.jemtechphoto.com

POSTCARDS

Pre-formatted

Paper Direct	800-272-7377
Viking	800-421-1222

Custom

US Press	912-244-5634
Color for Real Estate	800-221-1220
Modern Postcard	800-959-8365
Web Cards	www.web-cards.com

RADIO/TV

Radio & Television Interview Report	800-989-1400 ext.110 www.rtir.com
Yearbook of Experts, Authorities and Spokespersons	2233 Wisconsin Ave. NW Washington, DC 20007 1-800-Yearbook
Gale Directory of Publishing & Broadcast Media	Gale Research 835 Penobscot Bldg. 645 Griswold St. Detroit, MI 48226-4094
Radio and Records	www.rronline.com
Joe Sabah's Hot to Get on Radio and Talk Shows All Across America	Jsabah@aol.com 303-722-7200

STICKERS

Viking	800-421-1222
Interstate Label Co.	800-426-3261
Stephen Fossler Co.	800-762-0030